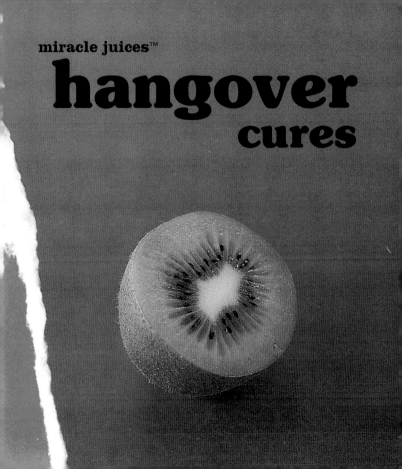

miracle juices™

# hangover
## cures

**Safety Note**

*Hangover Cures* should not be considered a replacement for professional medical treatment; a physician should be consulted on all matters relating to health. While the advice and information in this book is believed to be accurate, the publisher cannot accept any legal responsibility or liability for any injury or illness sustained while following the advice in this book.

First published in Great Britain in 2002 by Hamlyn,
a division of Octopus Publishing Group Ltd
2–4 Heron Quays, London E14 4JP

Copyright © Octopus Publishing Group Ltd 2002

Distributed in the United States and Canada by
Sterling Publishing Co., Inc.
387 Park Avenue South, New York, NY 10016-8810

ISBN 0 600 60672 4

A CIP catalogue record for this book is available
from the British Library

Printed and bound in China

10 9 8 7 6 5 4 3 2 1

# Contents

# introduction

### What is a hangover?

Alcohol can have a positive effect on our mood, sensations and behaviour, and for most of us a moderate amount reduces our inhibitions and encourages social interactions. In fact, one or two glasses of good red wine each day are thought to have health benefits and actually guard against heart disease. So, if it's so good, why do you feel so lousy?

Your head is throbbing, you feel dizzy, your mouth feels as dry as the Sahara and you think you might be sick again. The answer is simple. You've overdone it. Welcome to Hangover Land.

By sticking to a couple of units of alcohol (two small cans of beer, two glasses of wine or two measures of spirits), or by alternating an alcoholic drink with a drink of water, you would be feeling a lot better right now. Admittedly, alcohol tolerance differs greatly from person to person, but, whatever your level, many people enjoy the temporary euphoria that alcohol brings so much that they

### overindulgence

Worryingly, alcoholism affects one in ten people in the Western world. Those who drink to excess are putting themselves at risk from the following conditions:

- Stomach ulcers
- Colitis
- Decreased energy
- Liver, pancreas and gastrointestinal problems
- Short-term memory loss

forget about the potential effects on their health and the morning-after-the-night-before feeling that inevitably follows.

## How juices can help

When you have a hangover, the first thing you must do to feel human again is raise your blood sugar level. A fresh juice provides the quickest hit your body could receive of simple sugars which are easy to swallow and simple for your delicate system to digest. They also contain a fair quantity of water to help combat dehydration. Because they are made from raw fresh fruits and vegetables, juices also contain many vitamins and other nutrients which will help you on your way to a quick recovery.

# why you feel so bad

Although alcohol may seem to be a stimulant, essentially it acts as a depressant, slowing down the speed of all body functions including muscle contractions, reaction time, digestion and the thought process. It also drains the body of many essential nutrients.

As well as making you feel dehydrated, alcohol also places great strain on the liver, which works hard to neutralize the effects of drinking by breaking down the components of the alcohol.

If you eat a decent meal while drinking, or have only one alcoholic drink every hour throughout the evening with glasses of water in between to dilute the effect, the liver can perform its task effectively. But if the drinking is sustained and excessive, the liver will start to suffer. It will not be able to detoxify the body, as it will no longer be able to decompose glucose and fat or metabolize the alcohol.

There are many nutrients that can help the liver detoxify, but their action is impaired by the alcohol – for example, alcohol makes the liver expel all its folic acid into the bloodstream.

This causes a deficiency of folic acid, which is needed to work with vitamin B12 to stimulate the formation of red blood cells. Reduce the levels of one of those nutrients and the whole cycle is compromised. This is why you look so pale with a hangover.

## hangover hints

- Never drink coffee to sober yourself up. It is a diuretic that will deplete your body of fluids and make the alcohol even more concentrated.
- Don't drink grapefruit juice with alcohol as it increases its toxicity.
- Drink at least three glasses of water before going to bed.
- If you have vomited because of drinking, stop. Your body has had enough and your liver is in shock.
- Remember it only takes 20 minutes for alcohol to have an effect, and over an hour for the body to process each unit. Try to alternate each drink with a glass of water.
- Take 500 mg of milk thistle, 2 g of evening primrose oil, 1 g of vitamin C and a B complex vitamin before going out and drinking alcohol. Repeat in the morning. You may just avoid that hangover.

# vital hangover cure nutrients

| Nutrient | Actions | Good Source | Recommended daily dosage |
|----------|---------|-------------|--------------------------|
| **Vitamin A** | Vital for reducing susceptibility to infection by maintaining mucous membranes; antioxidant; essential for good digestion. | Found in milk, cheese, butter, eggs, meat, fish liver oil. Beta-carotene (converted into vitamin A in the body) found in yellow or deep orange fruits and vegetables such as cantaloupe melons and butternut squash, or leafy green vegetables such as spinach and broccoli. | 5000 iu for men, 4000 iu for women, 2000 iu for children |
| **Vitamin B1** | Involved in converting glucose into energy; prevents build-up of fatty deposits on artery walls; maintains a healthy nervous system. | Brewer's yeast, wheatgerm, whole grains, blackstrap molasses, soya beans, sunflower seeds, egg yolks, meat, fish, poultry, chickpeas. | 1.5 mg, although 50–60 mg can be taken safely when B1 has been severely depleted. |
| **Vitamin B12** | Works closely with folic acid in cell division; aids the absorption of vitamin A; vital for normal metabolism of nerve tissue; makes iron function better in the body; protects the liver from toxic substances. | Fish, dairy products, offal, eggs, beef, pork, tofu, spirulina, grains, yeast. | 2 mcg |
| **Vitamin C** | Powerful antioxidant; reduces allergic reactions; helps to form red blood cells; vital for healthy adrenal function. | Citrus fruits, all black and red berries, papaya, tomatoes, kiwi fruits, broccoli, cantaloupe melons, red peppers, cabbage, mango. | The minimum is 60 mg, but during times of stress increase this to 1–2 g per day, divided into two doses. |

| Nutrient | Actions | Good Source | Recommended daily dosage |
|----------|---------|-------------|--------------------------|
| **Vitamin D** | Aids in the absorption of calcium from the intestinal tract; guards against kidney disease. It is stored in the liver. | Oily fish, fortified milk, egg yolks, fish liver oils, offal, dairy products. | 400 iu |
| **Folic acid** | Necessary for the formation of red blood cells; brain function; aids the function of the liver. | Spinach, asparagus, Brussels sprouts, soya beans, root vegetables, brewer's yeast, whole grains, wheatgerm. | 400–800 mcg |
| **Selenium** | Antioxidant; necessary for production of prostaglandins, which affect blood pressure; has a detoxifying effect on heavy metals, smoke, drugs, alcohol and peroxidized fats. | Brewer's yeast, wheatgerm, whole grains, sesame seeds, sunflower seeds, Brazil nuts, seafood, cabbage, broccoli, cucumber, garlic, onions, radishes. | 50–200 mcg |
| **Potassium** | Stimulates kidneys to excrete toxic waste; regulates neuromuscular activity in conjunction with calcium; oxygenates the brain; regulates the fluid balance in the body with sodium. | All vegetables, oranges, whole grains, sunflower seeds, mint leaves, potatoes, garlic, brewer's yeast, brown rice, blackstrap molasses, dates, dried fruit, bananas, tomatoes, pineapple. | 2000 mg |

# why juice?

Vital vitamins and minerals such as antioxidants, vitamins A, B, C and E, folic acid, potassium, calcium, magnesium, zinc and amino acids are present in fresh fruits and vegetables, and are all necessary for optimum health. Because juicing removes the indigestible fibre in fruits and vegetables, the nutrients are available to the body in much larger quantities than if the piece of fruit or vegetable were eaten whole. For example, when you eat a raw carrot you are able to assimilate only about 1 per cent of the available beta-carotene, because many of the nutrients are trapped in the fibre. When a carrot is juiced, thereby removing the fibre, nearly 100 per cent of the beta-carotene can be assimilated. Juicing several types of fruits and vegetables on a daily basis is therefore an easy way to ensure that your body receives its full quota of vitamins and minerals.

In addition, fruits and vegetables provide another substance absolutely essential for good health — water. Most people don't consume enough water. In fact, many of the fluids we drink — coffee, tea, soft drinks, alcoholic beverages and artificially flavoured drinks — contain substances that require extra water for the body to eliminate, and tend to be dehydrating. Fruit and vegetable juices are free of these unnecessary substances.

## Your health

A diet high in fruits and vegetables can prevent and help to cure a wide range of ailments. At the cutting edge of nutritional research are the plant chemicals known as phytochemicals, which hold the key to preventing deadly diseases such as cancer and heart disease, and others such as asthma, arthritis and allergies.

Although juicing benefits your overall health, it should be used only to complement your daily eating plan. You must still eat enough from the other food groups (such as grains, dairy food and pulses) to ensure your body maintains strong bones and healthy cells. If you are following a specially prescribed diet, or are under medical supervision, do discuss any drastic changes with your health practitioner before beginning any type of new health regime.

# how to juice

Available in a variety of models, juicers work by separating the fruit and vegetable juice from the pulp. Choose a juicer with a reputable brand name, that has an opening big enough for larger fruits and vegetables, and make sure it is easy to take apart and clean, otherwise you may become discouraged from using it.

## Types of juicer

A citrus juicer or lemon squeezer is ideal for extracting the juice from oranges, lemons, limes and grapefruit, especially if you want to add just a small amount of citrus juice to another liquid. Pure citrus juice has a high acid content, which may upset your stomach, so it is best diluted.

Centrifugal juicers are the most widely used and affordable juicers available. Fresh fruits and vegetables are fed into a rapidly spinning grater, and the pulp separated from the juice by centrifugal force. The pulp is retained in the machine while the juice runs into a separate jug. A centrifugal juicer produces less juice than the more expensive masticating juicer, which works by pulverizing fruits and vegetables, and pushing them through a wire mesh with immense force.

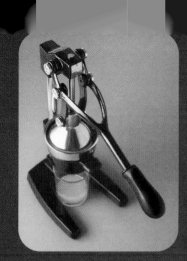

to two parts water will lessen any staining produced by the fruits and vegetables.

## Preparing produce for juicing

It is best to prepare ingredients just before juicing so that fewer nutrients are lost through oxidization. Cut or tear foods into manageable pieces for juicing. If the ingredients are not organic, do not include stems, skins or roots, but if the produce is organic, you can put everything in the juicer. However, don't include the skins from pineapple, mango, papaya, citrus fruit and banana, and remove the stones from avocados, apricots, peaches, mangoes and plums. You can include melon seeds, particularly watermelon, as these are full of juice. For grape juice, choose green grapes with an amber tinge or black grapes with a darkish bloom. Leave the pith on lemons for the pectin content.

## Cleaning the juicer

Clean your juicing machine thoroughly, as any residue left may harbour bacterial growth — a toothbrush or nailbrush works well for removing stubborn residual pulp. Leaving the equipment to soak in warm, soapy water will loosen the residue from those hard-to-reach places. A solution made up of one part white vinegar

**13**

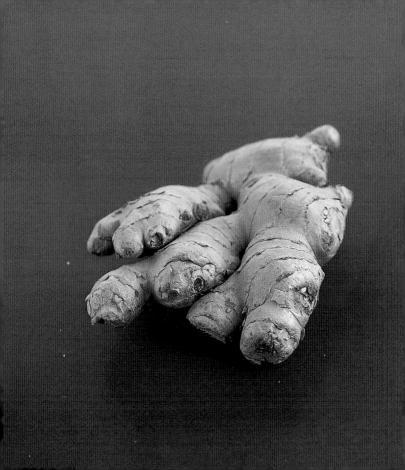

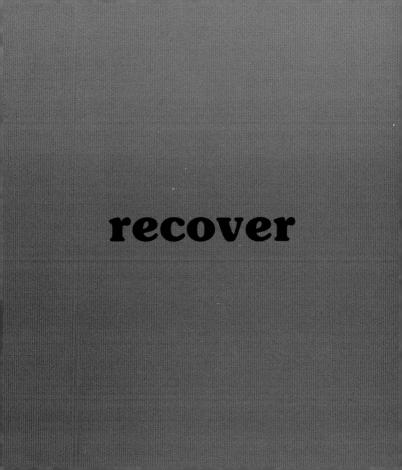

recover

If you ache from head to toe and can't seem to function, you need to replace vital potassium, get some vitamin C into your system and could probably benefit from some extra B vitamins. This fruity smoothie is high in potassium, but if you really want to boost the vitamin content, add a spoonful of blackstrap molasses or powdered spirulina. Both of these are high in B1 while spirulina is also a good source of B12. They will change the taste quite dramatically, but if you are feeling that bad it will be worth it.

# acher shaker

100 g (3½ oz)
   strawberries
300 g (10 oz) pineapple
1 banana
ice cubes

Juice the strawberries and pineapple. Pour the juice into a blender or food processor, add the banana and a couple of ice cubes and process. Serve and sip slowly through a straw.

**Makes 300 ml (½ pint)**

## Nutritional Values

- Kcals: 289
- vitamin C: 119 mg
- magnesium: 87 mg
- potassium: 961 mg

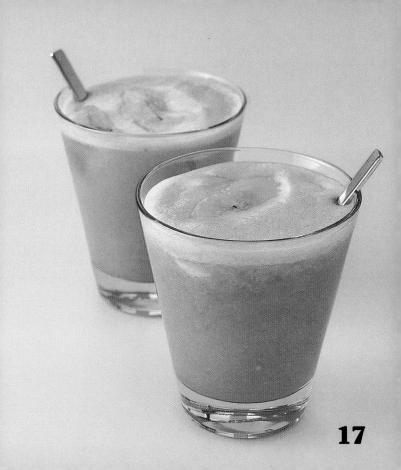

**17**

Ginger will help to alleviate symptoms of nausea, and carrot and apple provide a burst of nutrients.

# pick-me-up

**200 g (7 oz) carrots**
**1 tart-flavoured apple,**
**such as Granny Smith**
**1 cm (½ inch) piece of**
**fresh root ginger**
**ice cubes**

Scrub the carrots and wash the apple. Cut the carrots, apple and ginger into even-sized pieces and juice. Pour into a glass and add a couple of ice cubes.
**Makes 250 ml (8 fl oz)**

## Nutritional Values

- Kcals: 127
- vitamin A: 60833 iu
- vitamin C: 30 mg
- iron: 0.9 mg
- calcium: 59 mg

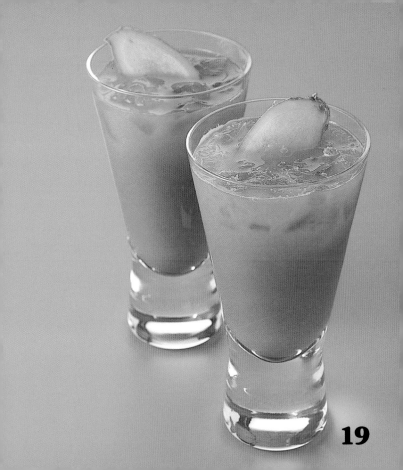

19

When you have given your liver a severe thrashing, it is going to need help to rid itself of toxins and get on with metabolizing glucose to provide you with energy. The ingredients in this juice are excellent detoxifiers and also give a kick to the immune system. The taste is quite bitter, but the juice is very effective. Liquidizing the juice with ice helps to make it more palatable.

# upbeet

**100 g (3½ oz) celeriac**
**50 g (2 oz) beetroot**
**100 g (3½ oz) carrots**
**50 g (2 oz) radicchio**
**1 apple**
**ice cubes**

Peel the celeriac, scrub the beetroot and carrots and cut them into sticks. Juice all the ingredients, then process the juice in a blender or food processor with a couple of ice cubes.

**Makes 200 ml (7 fl oz)**

## Nutritional Values

- Kcals: 191
- vitamin A: 27102 iu
- potassium: 1033 mg
- selenium: 2.3 mcg

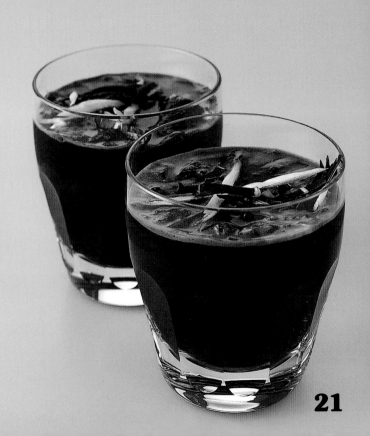

The cucumber will help to flush out the kidneys and the grapefruit aids
the elimination of toxins, both vital for hangover relief and recovery.

# lemon aid

**600 g (1 lb 4 oz)
grapefruit
750 g (1½ lb) cucumber
1 lemon
ice cubes
sparkling mineral water**

Juice the grapefruit, cucumber and lemon.
Pour into a jug over ice, and top up with
sparkling mineral water. Decorate with
chopped mint and slices of cucumber
and lemon, if liked.

**Makes 400 ml (14 fl oz)**

*To decorate:*
**chopped mint
cucumber slices
lemon slices**

## Nutritional Values

- Kcals: 302
- vitamin C: 273 mg
- potassium: 1627 mg
- magnesium: 132 mg
- zinc: 1.9 mg

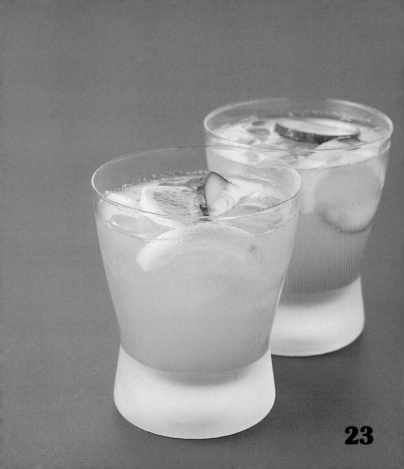

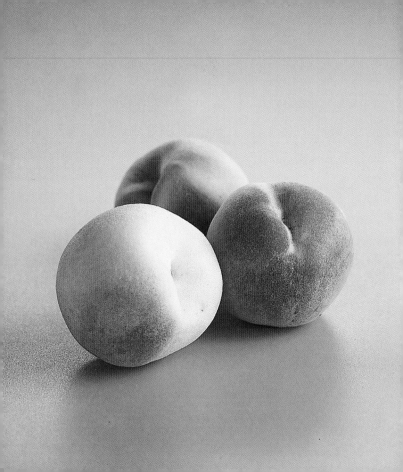

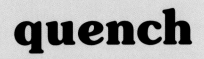

quench

As well as freshening your breath, mint is a good source of potassium. When combined with celeriac and celery, it helps to replenish potassium supplies that have been lost through frequent urination caused by alcohol.

# gargle
# blaster

100 g (3½ oz) celeriac
100 g (3½ oz) Jerusalem
   artichokes
100 g (3½ oz) celery
small bunch of mint
ice cubes

Peel the celeriac and chop it into sticks; scrub the artichokes. Juice the vegetables and the mint, being sure to alternate the mint leaves with the other ingredients to prevent the juicer getting clogged up. Process the juice in a blender or food processor with a couple of ice cubes and serve.

**Makes 200 ml (7 fl oz)**

## Nutritional Values

- Kcals: 130
- vitamin C: 21 g
- potassium: 632 mg

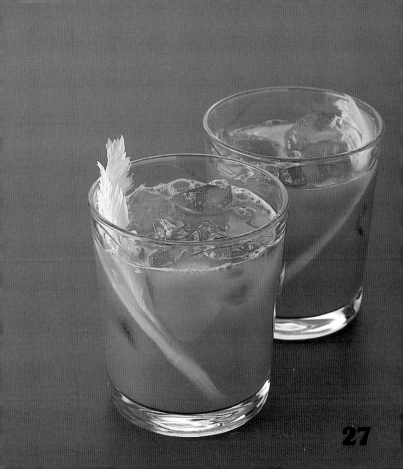

Peach has an alkalizing effect on the digestive system, while ginger works wonders for nausea and honey also helps settle a queasy stomach.

# peach fizz

**250 g (8 oz) peaches**
**2.5 cm (1 inch) cube**
   **fresh root ginger,**
   **roughly chopped**
**sparkling mineral water**
**mint leaves**

Juice the peach and ginger and serve in a tall glass over ice, with a splash of sparkling water and a couple of mint leaves. Sip slowly to calm your stomach.
**Makes 200 ml (7 fl oz)**

## Nutritional Values

- Kcals: 127
- vitamin C: 10 mg
- potassium: 390 mg

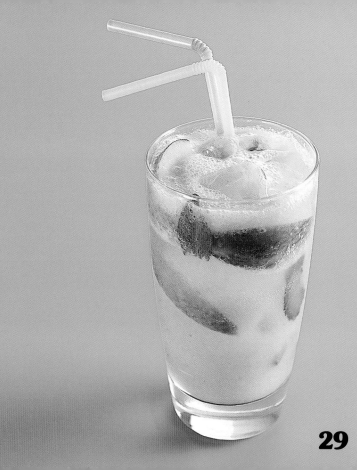

**29**

Not only is lettuce calming to an aching head, it also is a great source of vitamin A and potassium. Another beneficial effect is that it eases excess gas. If your liver is really feeling the strain, substitute the calming effects of chamomile tea for the detoxifying powers of dandelion leaf tea.

# mind
# bath

**100 g (3½ oz)
  Romaine lettuce
½ lemon, peeled
100 ml (3½ fl oz)
  chilled chamomile tea
ice cubes
lemon slice**

Juice the lettuce and lemon then mix with the chilled chamomile tea. Serve in a tall glass over ice with a slice of lemon.
**Makes 200 ml (7 fl oz)**

## Nutritional Values

- Kcals: 24
- vitamin A: 3000 iu
- potassium: 518 mg

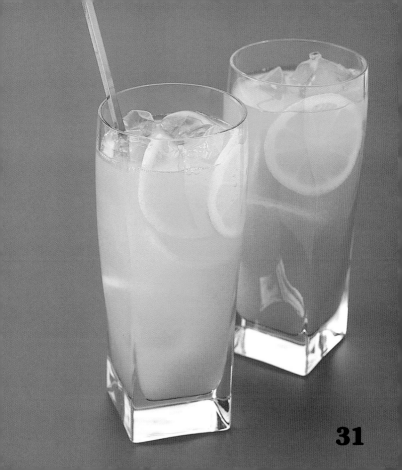

This rich and sweet juice is a great blood restorer and liver regenerator. This is very important after a hangover because if the liver has been overtaxed, it won't be able to cleanse and purify the blood effectively, leaving the blood full of potentially harmful toxins.

# live wire

**100 g (3½ oz) red grapes**
**100 g (3½ oz) beetroot**
**100 g (3½ oz) plums**
**ice cubes**

Juice the grapes, beetroot and plums and serve in a tumbler over ice.

**Makes 200 ml (7 fl oz)**

## Nutritional Values

- Kcals: 143
- vitamin C: 15.3 mg
- potassium: 611 mg
- folic acid: 51 mcg

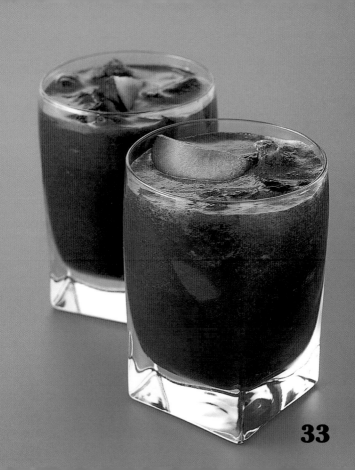

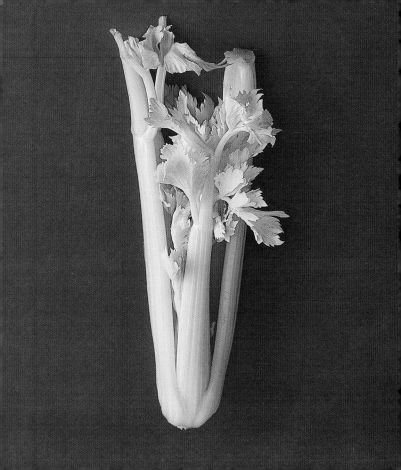

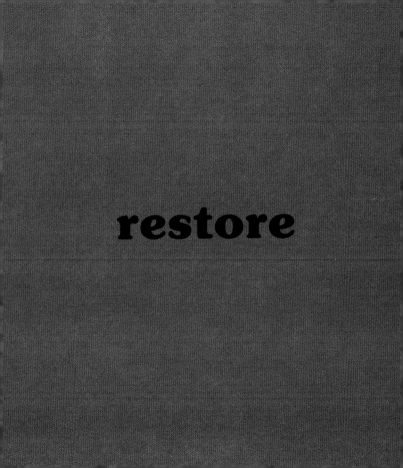

restore

If you want to cleanse and rehydrate your system, melon has a fantastically high water content and replenishes lost fluids very quickly, particularly when taken on its own. Cantaloupe melon contains high levels of beta-carotene, vitamin C and potassium. Juice it with the seeds for extra trace elements.

# morning glory

**500 g (1 lb) cantaloupe melon, peeled, or any melon flesh and seeds**
**ice cubes**

Juice the melon then serve over ice. Drink immediately.
**Makes 300 ml (½ pint)**

## Nutritional Values

- Kcals: 180
- vitamin A: 15474 iu
- vitamin C: 214 g
- potassium: 1482 mg
- folic acid: 81 mcg

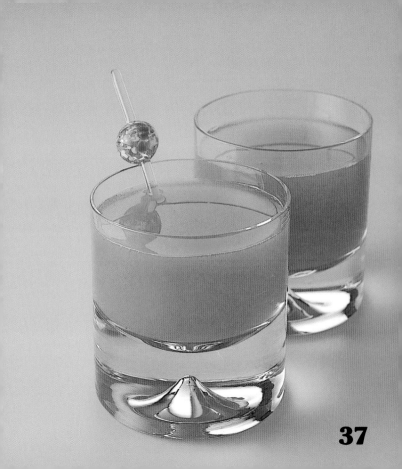

Because of their high potassium content, both carrot and fennel are effective detoxifiers and good for restoring fluid balance. Fennel also helps to digest fats, which will give a bit of a help to your overworked liver. A glass of this juice should give you an immediate lift and ensure that the whites of your eyes are white, not bloodshot.

# eye opener

**200 g (7 oz) carrots**
**200 g (7 oz) fennel**
**ice cubes**

Juice the carrots and fennel.
Serve the juice in a tall glass over ice.
**Makes 200 ml (7 fl oz)**

## Nutritional Values

- Kcals: 152
- vitamin A: 61027 iu
- potassium: 1527 mg
- selenium: 3.3 mcg

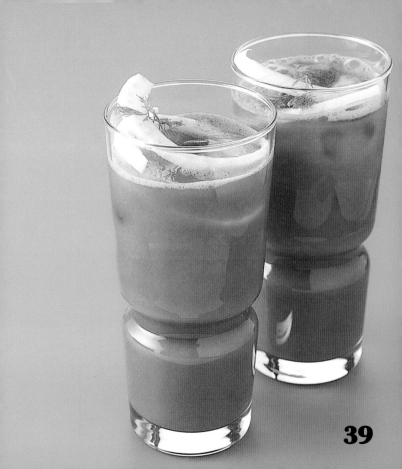

**39**

If you want to ensure thorough cleansing of your kidneys, liver and digestive tract, this juice is superb. Cauliflower helps to purify the blood; it lowers blood pressure and is a great antioxidant, but it does taste a little on the strong side. It is also a great source of folic acid and one of the best things you could possibly have to boost a flagging immune system. If you have a sweet tooth, add an apple to soften the flavour.

# veg out

100 g (3½ oz) cauliflower
200 g (7 oz) carrots
1 large tomato
ice cubes

Juice the cauliflower, carrots and tomato. Serve over ice if desired.

**Makes 200 ml (7 fl oz)**

## Nutritional Values

- Kcals: 139
- vitamin A: 62153 iu
- vitamin C: 113 mg
- potassium: 1309 mg
- folic acid: 108 mcg

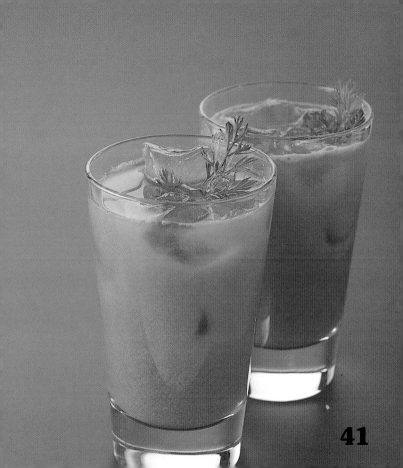

If you are feeling really dehydrated, you are going to need more than just a glass of water. To feel better, you will also need to replace the vital nutrients you have lost. Your liver will have expelled its entire store of folic acid into the bloodstream to be excreted in the urine along with vitamin C and potassium. This juice will give you back some of what you need and help to quench that insatiable thirst.

# the rehydrator

1 orange
50 g (2 oz) cucumber
100 ml (3½ fl oz)
   cranberry juice
ice cubes

Peel the orange, leaving on as much pith as possible. Juice the orange and cucumber. Mix the juice with the cranberry juice and serve in a tall glass over ice.
**Makes 200 ml (7 fl oz)**

## Nutritional Values

- Kcals: 119
- vitamin C: 106 mg
- potassium: 328 mg
- folic acid: 48 mcg

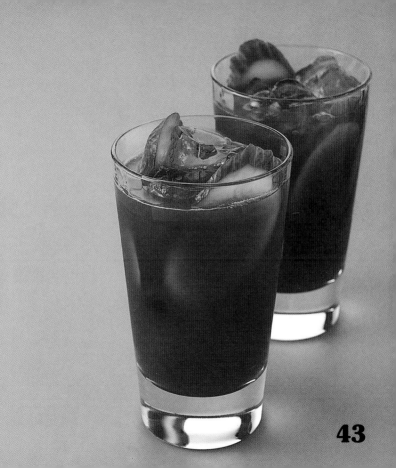

**43**

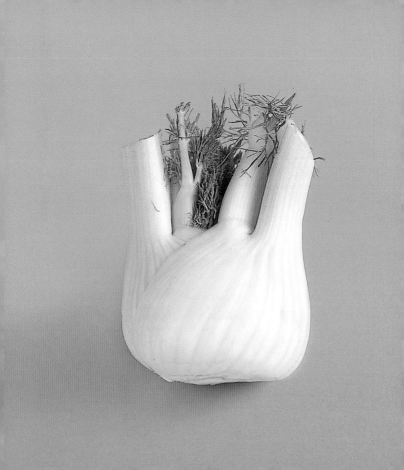

# awaken

If you have woken up to find that your body has gone into toxic overload, with blocked sinuses and a heavy head, then this is the ideal juice for you. Radishes are a great expectorant and will help to dissolve mucous. Carrots contain huge amounts of vitamin A, which is vital for healthy mucous membranes and fighting infection. Apples help remove toxins and restore beneficial bacteria to your toxin-ridden digestive system.

# clear ahead

**250 g (8 oz) carrots**
**50 g (2 oz) radishes**
**1 large apple**
**ice cubes**

Juice the carrots, radishes and apple. Pour the juice into a blender or food processor and process with a couple of ice cubes.
**Makes 200 ml (7 fl oz)**

## Nutritional Values

- Kcals: 178
- vitamin A: 60838 iu
- vitamin C: 38 g
- potassium: 962 mg
- selenium: 2.7 mcg

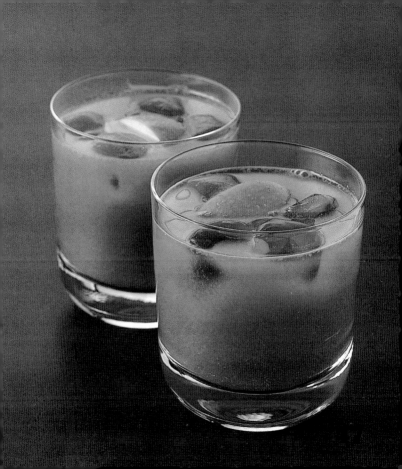

This is a super juice, especially if you've had a few too many cocktails. Broccoli is one of the greatest all-round foods, as it is rich in vitamins C and A, magnesium, folic acid and selenium; it is a great antioxidant and stimulates the liver. Spinach has very high levels of vitamin A, folic acid, magnesium and potassium, and will give the immune system a real kick. Finally, apples are superb detoxifiers.

# hangover express

**150 g (5 oz) broccoli**
**2 apples**
**150 g (5 oz) spinach**
**ice cubes (optional)**

Juice the broccoli, apples and spinach, alternating the spinach leaves with the broccoli and apple to ensure that the machine doesn't get clogged up with the leaves. This juice has a green but very sweet taste, so blend it with a couple of ice cubes before serving, if you wish.

**Makes 200 ml (7 fl oz)**

## Nutritional Values

- Kcals: 230
- vitamin A: 18948 iu
- vitamin C: 162 g
- magnesium: 155 mg
- potassium: 1527 mg
- selenium: 2.5 mcg
- folic acid: 270 mcg

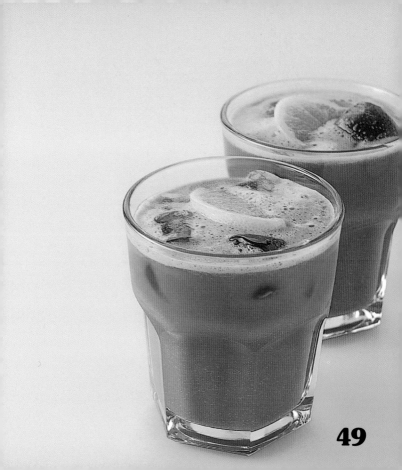

If your kidneys were aching when you woke up, give them a good flush with this extra-light refreshing juice. The pectin in the pear will aid the removal of toxins, while cranberries are renowned for killing bacteria and viruses in the kidneys, bladder and urinary tract.

# hazy days

1 large pear
100 ml (3½ fl oz)
  cranberry juice
ice cubes

Juice the pear and mix the pear juice with the cranberry juice. Serve in a tall glass over ice.

**Makes 200 ml (7 fl oz)**

## Nutritional Values

- Kcals: 153
- vitamin A: 468 iu
- vitamin C: 39 mg
- potassium: 242 mg

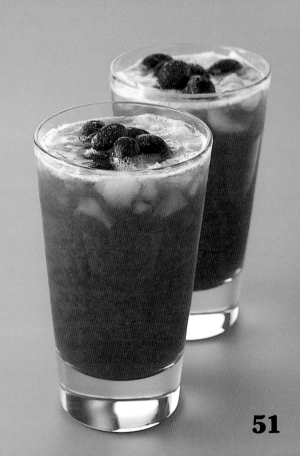

Remember that kiwi fruits contain even more vitamin C than oranges, so by combining the two fruits you are giving yourself an even more potent dose. Add to that high levels of potassium and folic acid, and watch that hangover fade away.

# c double

**2 large oranges**
**2 kiwi fruits**
**(skins left on)**
**ice cubes**
**lemon twist**
**mint sprig**

Peel the oranges, leaving on as much pith as possible, and juice them along with the kiwi fruits. Serve over ice.
**Makes 200 ml (7 fl oz)**

## Nutritional Values

- Kcals: 216
- vitamin A: 806 iu
- vitamin C: 290 mg
- potassium: 974 mg
- folic acid: 80 mcg

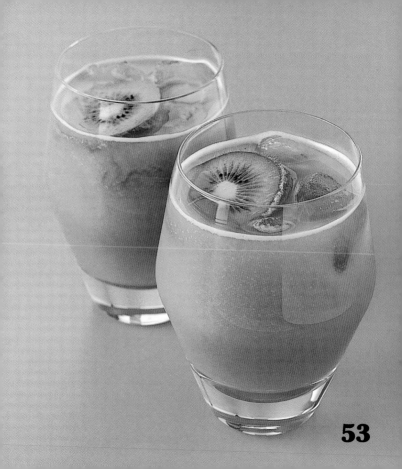

**53**

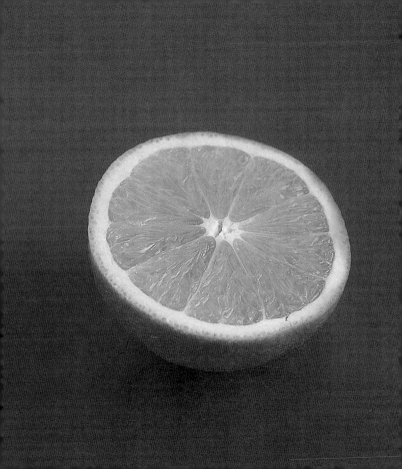

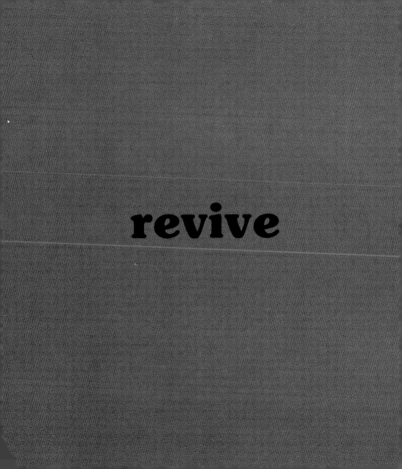

revive

Tomatoes and carrots provide large amounts of vitamin C to replenish lost supplies. Garlic, ginger and horseradish are all powerful antioxidants - imperative for fighting off infections.

# hot stuff

300 g (10 oz) tomatoes
100 g (3½ oz) celery
2.5 cm (1 inch) cube
   fresh root ginger,
   roughly chopped
1 garlic clove
2.5 cm (1 inch) cube
   fresh horseradish
175 g (6 oz) carrots
ice cubes
celery slivers,
   to decorate (optional)

Juice all the ingredients, process the juice with a couple of ice cubes in a blender or food processor and serve in a tumbler. Decorate with celery slivers, if desired.
**Makes 150 ml (¼ pint)**

## Nutritional Values

- Kcals: 189
- vitamin A: 51253 iu
- vitamin C: 87 mg
- selenium: 4.47 mcg
- zinc: 5.52 mg

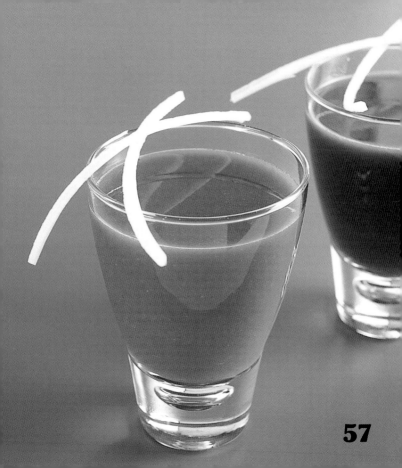

If you can't lift your head off the pillow because it is throbbing so badly, and you are feeling the effects of a late-night curry, you will find this juice brilliant. Celery helps flush out aggravating toxins and rehydrate the system, while the fennel helps to digest fat and will give your liver a break; grapefruit is a powerful blood cleanser.

# mother nature

½ **grapefruit, peeled**
**100 g (3½ oz) celery**
**100 g (3½ oz) fennel**
**ice cubes**

Juice the grapefruit, celery and fennel and serve in a tall glass over ice.
**Makes 200 ml (7 fl oz)**

## Nutritional Values

- Kcals: 87
- vitamin C: 54 mg
- potassium: 729 mg
- folic acid: 28 mcg

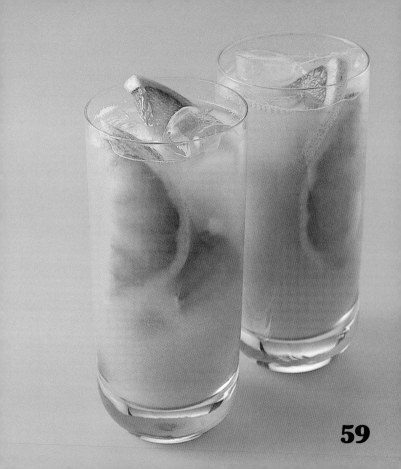

**59**

The three ingredients in this juice are key players in blood cleansing and will help you to lose that sluggish feeling. Cabbage is at its most powerful when raw, as it detoxifies the stomach and upper colon, improves digestion, stimulates the immune system, kills bacteria and viruses, and is a natural antioxidant. Tomatoes are very effective for reducing liver inflammation and, because they are alkaline, they should help if you have a queasy stomach. Parsley is also alkaline and acts as an anticoagulant. It also has the added benefit of freshening breath.

# raw energy

**100 g (3½ oz) tomatoes**
**200 g (7 oz) cabbage**
**large handful of parsley**
**celery stick (optional)**

Juice the tomatoes, cabbage and parsley and serve in a tumbler. Add sliced tomatoes or a stick of celery, if you like.
**Makes 200 ml (7 fl oz)**

## Nutritional Values

- Kcals: 77
- vitamin A: 6858 iu
- vitamin C: 133 mg
- potassium: 825 mg
- folic acid: 155 mcg

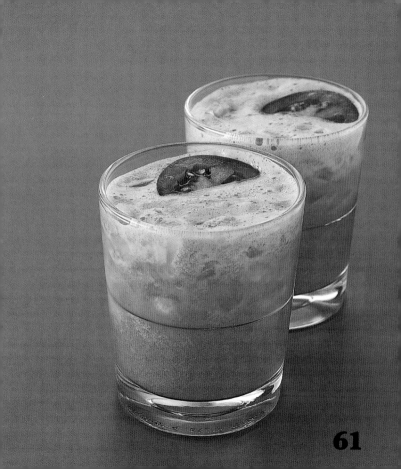

Papaya helps to calm the digestive system, cucumber flushes out toxins and orange gives a great boost of vitamin C. The overall effect is calming and rehydrating.

# morning after

**125 g (4 oz) papaya**
**2 oranges**
**125 g (4 oz) cucumber**
**ice cubes**

*To decorate*
**cucumber slices**
**papaya slices**

Peel the papaya and the oranges (leaving as much of the pith as possible) and wash the cucumber. Juice them together and serve in a tall glass over ice. Decorate with slices of cucumber and papaya.
**Makes 200 ml (7 fl oz)**

## Nutritional Values

- Kcals: 184
- vitamin A: 1123 iu
- vitamin C: 218 mg
- magnesium: 51 mg
- potassium: 1004 mg
- selenium: 2 mcg

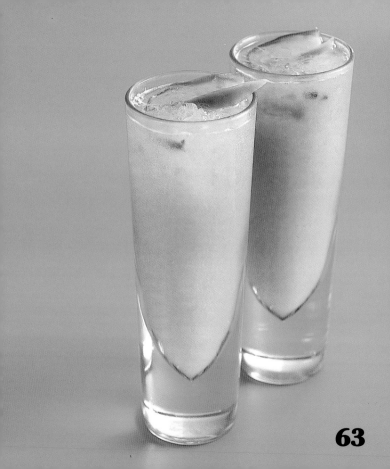

**63**

# index

# acknowledgements

The publisher would like to thank The Juicer Company for the loan of the Champion juicer and the Orange X citrus juicer (featured on pages 12 and 13).

**The Juicer Company**
**28 Shambles**
**York**
**YO1 7LX**
**Tel: (01904) 541541**
**www.thejuicercompany.co.uk**

**Executive Editor** Nicola Hill
**Editor** Camilla James
**Executive Art Editor** Geoff Fennell
**Designer** Sue Michniewicz
**Senior Production Controller** Jo Sim
**Photographer** Stephen Conroy
**Home Economist** David Morgan
**Stylist** Angela Swaffield
All photographs © Octopus Publishing Group Ltd